WEIGHT LOSS BOOK FOR WOMEN OVER 40

"A well detailed guide to loosing excess weight"

TIM BROWN

TABLE OF CONTENT

INTRODUCTION

Welcome to the Journey: Recognizing the Particular Difficulties in Losing Weight for Women Over 40

Starting a weight reduction journey is a complex undertaking for a woman over 40. You may have seen that losing those excess pounds is more complicated than it was when you were younger. A sluggish metabolism, hormonal fluctuations, and a host of other issues might make reaching your weight reduction objectives seem unattainable. But it's crucial to keep in mind that you're not going through this alone.

This book is a thorough manual designed primarily to address the particular difficulties with weight reduction that women over 40 have. It seeks to provide you with the information, resources, and techniques needed to traverse this phase of life effectively. We will explore the complexities of the mind-body connection, hormonal changes, and the effects of ageing on metabolism in order to establish a comprehensive and long-lasting strategy for weight control.

This book combines scientific data, valuable tips, and motivating insights to assist you in creating a customized strategy that meets your objectives and way of life. These guidelines may be customized to meet your own goals, whether your goal is to lose a substantial amount of weight or to feel better overall.

Keep in mind that this journey is about more than simply losing weight; it's also about adopting a healthy lifestyle and developing a good connection with your body. It's about developing resilience, self-love, and empowerment that goes beyond scale numbers.

In order to achieve long-term success, we will examine different facets of diet, exercise, mental health, and sustainable lifestyle modifications with each chapter. We will also highlight the value of stress reduction, self-care, and the assistance of others in your weight loss endeavors.

So, let's go off on this life-changing journey together. Let's arm ourselves with the information and resources needed to meet the following challenges. Let's celebrate each accomplishment and stride forward, understanding that every attempt is an indication of your grit and tenacity.

Now is the beginning of your path to a better, healthier, and more satisfying existence. Together, we can turn it into a voyage of self-awareness, empowerment, and enduring well-being wellbeing.

CHAPTER 1: Foundations for Successful Weight Loss

Adopting the Mind-Body Link: Developing the Appropriate Mentality for Prolonged Achievement

Maintaining general well-being requires accepting the mind-body link, comprehending the biology of ageing, and taking stock of one's health, particularly for women over 40. Hormonal balance often shifts significantly at this period of life, which may have an impact on a number of body processes, including metabolism, weight control, and general health. Through the development of an appropriate mentality and knowledge of physiological changes, women may take charge of their health, lower their risks, and design customized programs that will support their long-term prosperity and well-being.

The complex interrelationship between psychological and physical health is known as the "mind-body connection." Long-term success requires the appropriate mentality, particularly for women over 40 who may be going through a variety of life changes, such as hormonal changes and physiological transitions. Women may promote a holistic approach to health that incorporates mental, emotional, and physical well-being by accepting the mind-body link. This might include self-care techniques that support a robust and healthy attitude, such as yoga, mindfulness meditation, cognitive behavioral therapy, and other types of self-care. This attitude builds resilience and improves general well-being by emphasizing positive self-image, realistic goal-setting, and the development of a feeling of satisfaction and purpose.

How Hormonal Changes Affect Weight Loss after 40: Understanding the Biology of Aging

Hormonal fluctuations are a significant contributor to ageing in women over 40 and may have an impact on many areas of health, including weight control. Hormonal shifts, especially in estrogen and progesterone levels, may cause metabolic alterations, increased fat storage, and reduced muscle mass throughout perimenopause and menopause, making weight reduction more difficult. Comprehending the effects of these hormonal shifts is essential to formulating practical plans for preserving a healthy weight and general well-being. A well-rounded, nutrient-dense diet, consistent exercise, strength training, and stress-reduction methods may all help lessen the impact of hormone fluctuations and promote long-term weight control.

Evaluating Your Health: Recognizing Possible Hazards and Developing a Customized Strategy for Women Over 40

In order to identify possible dangers and create a customized strategy to improve the well-being of women over 40, it is imperative that one first assess their health. Frequent screenings for health issues, such as blood pressure, cholesterol, bone density, and breast health, may aid in the early detection of health issues and allow for prompt action. Furthermore, evaluating lifestyle elements, including nutrition, exercise, sleep habits, and stress levels, is crucial to comprehending their influence on general health and well-being. Maintaining optimum health and lowering the risk of age-related health disorders may be significantly aided by developing a tailored health plan that includes regular exercise, a balanced diet, stress management strategies, enough sleep, and preventative health measures

In summation, the core tenets of fostering long-term success and well-being for women over 40 include:

- Accepting the mind-body link.
- Comprehending the biology of ageing.
- Evaluating one's health.

Through the promotion of a comprehensive health strategy, comprehension of the effects of hormonal fluctuations, and proactive mitigation of possible health hazards, women may enable themselves to have happy, healthy, and active lives as they mature.

Promoting optimum health and well-being requires developing a sustainable and balanced food plan, adding necessary nutrients and antioxidants, and putting into practice workable meal planning and portion management measures, particularly for women over 40. A well-crafted diet regimen that emphasizes nutrient-dense meals and sensible portion management may improve general health, energy levels, and vitality as the body experiences different changes with age, including hormone shifts and metabolic modifications.

CHAPTER 2: Navigating the Nutrition Maze

The Power of Nutrition: Creating a Balanced and Sustainable Diet

For women over 40, a balanced, sustainable food plan is crucial to their general health and well-being. A wide range of nutrient-dense foods, such as whole grains, lean meats, fruits, vegetables, and healthy fats, should be a part of such a strategy. It is essential to prioritize the consumption of whole, minimally processed foods while lowering the intake of processed foods, refined carbohydrates, and saturated fats in order to maintain a healthy weight, control hormonal fluctuations, and reduce the risk of age-related health issues. For women over 40, maintaining maximum health and vitality may be facilitated by following a well-rounded food plan that includes necessary fatty acids, vitamins, minerals, and appropriate water.

Superfoods for Women Over 40: Including Antioxidants and Vital Nutrients

For women over 40, including superfoods high in antioxidants and critical nutrients is crucial to supporting overall health and wellbeing. Superfoods are excellent sources of vital nutrients, such as vitamins, minerals, and antioxidants, which may help lower inflammation, enhance cognitive function, increase immunity, and encourage healthy ageing. Examples of these superfoods include berries, leafy greens, fatty fish, nuts, seeds, and whole grains. These nutrient-dense meals may also provide vital micronutrients, such as calcium, vitamin D, and omega-3 fatty acids, which are critical for heart health, muscular function, and bone health. These micronutrients may also become more significant as people age.

Meal Planning and Portion Control: Useful Techniques for Women Over 40 to Succeed in the Long Run

For women over 40 to maintain a healthy weight and promote overall well-being, it is essential to put into practice realistic meal planning and portion management measures.

Incorporating mindful eating techniques, such as portion control, anticipating feelings of hunger and fullness, and organizing balanced meals in advance, may promote weight management by preventing overeating. Measuring serving sizes, using smaller plates, and paying attention to portion sizes while dining out are practical tactics that encourage better eating practices and assist in long-term weight control. For women over 40, meal planning and portion management techniques may be made even more successful by including mindful eating and frequent physical exercise.

In conclusion, the key to promoting optimal health, well-being, and longevity for women over 40 is to create a sustainable and balanced diet plan, incorporate superfoods that are rich in vital nutrients and antioxidants, and put into practice realistic meal planning and portion control strategies. Women may improve their diet and lifestyle to promote healthy ageing and overall vitality by emphasizing nutrient-dense meals, portion management, and mindful eating habits.

CHAPTER 3: Crafting an Effective Exercise Regimen

Personalizing Your Exercise: Exercise Plans Designed for Women Over 40

A comprehensive fitness plan for women over 40 must include customized exercise regimens, strength training for metabolism and bone health, and focused physical activity to maximize cardiovascular health. Personalizing exercise regimens with an emphasis on cardiovascular health, flexibility, and strength training can help support overall fitness, promote bone health, increase metabolism, and improve cardiovascular function as the body changes with age. These changes include muscle loss, decreased bone density, and hormonal fluctuations.

To enhance general health and well-being, customized exercise regimens for women over 40 should include a mix of aerobic, strength, and flexibility exercises. It is essential to customize exercise regimens to each person's fitness level, preferences, and pre-existing health issues in order to maximize safety and efficacy. Exercises like Pilates, yoga, cycling, swimming, and brisk walking may help increase flexibility, strengthen the heart, and improve general health. Incorporating workouts that focus on specific muscle areas, such as the upper, lower, and core, may also help preserve muscle mass, improve balance, and assist in developing strength, all of which enhance general physical fitness and vitality.

Strength Training: Safe Ways to Gain Lean Muscle Mass and Improve Bone Health and Metabolism

For women over 40, strength exercise is crucial for maintaining lean muscle mass, boosting metabolism, and supporting bone health. Workouts, including weight bearing, resistance training, and bodyweight workouts, may promote general bone health, lower the risk of osteoporosis, and increase bone density. Exercises like lunges, squats, push-ups, and weightlifting with the correct resistance may help develop lean muscle mass and speed up metabolism, which can improve general physical function and weight control. When doing strength training activities, it is crucial to put appropriate technique, progressive development, and enough rest first in order to guarantee safety and efficacy.

Cardiovascular Health and Fat-Burning Activities: Optimizing Physical Activity's Advantages for Women Over 40

For women over 40, optimizing cardiovascular health via focused physical exercise is crucial to supporting heart health, enhancing overall well-being, and improving endurance. Walking, running, cycling, and swimming are examples of aerobic workouts that may strengthen the heart, enhance circulation, and improve cardiovascular health in general. Optimizing fat burning, raising metabolic rate, and supporting weight control may also be achieved by using circuit training, high-intensity exercises, and interval training. Women over 40 may attain ideal cardiovascular health and general fitness by making regular physical activity a priority, drinking enough water, and engaging in a range of cardiovascular exercises.

To sum up, increasing total fitness and well-being for women over 40 requires creating personalized exercise regimens, including strength training for metabolism and bone health, and optimizing cardiovascular health via focused physical activity. Women may improve bone health, metabolism, and cardiovascular function by concentrating on a well-rounded fitness regimen that incorporates strength training, aerobic conditioning, and flexibility exercises. This will eventually encourage a healthier and more active lifestyle as they age.

Maintaining general well-being and attaining long-term success requires overcoming obstacles and plateaus, developing good habits, and managing stress and sleep, particularly for women over 40. Age-related changes in the body include hormonal variations and metabolic alterations. To support weight control, promote general health, and cultivate a positive mentality, it is essential to successfully manage stress, incorporate good behaviors, and maintain motivation.

CHAPTER 4: Lifestyle Modifications for Sustainable Results

Handling Stress and Sleep: Revealing the Link between Rest and Loss of Weight

For women over 40, stress management and getting enough sleep are essential for supporting hormone balance, weight control, and general well-being. While getting too little sleep may interfere with energy levels, eating power, metabolism, and weight gain, high levels of stress can cause hormonal imbalances, increased cravings, and weight gain. Incorporating relaxation methods like yoga, meditation, and deep breathing exercises may assist healthy weight control, lower stress levels, and improve emotional well-being. For women over 40, excellent sleep quality, hormone balance, and general health may be achieved by establishing a regular sleep schedule, developing a calming nighttime ritual, and making sure their sleeping environment is pleasant.

Creating Healthier Routines: Including Long-Term Adjustments in Your Everyday Activities

For women over 40, developing healthy behaviors is crucial to promoting both long-term success and general well-being. Making long-lasting adjustments to everyday routines—like eating a balanced diet, often exercising, giving self-care priority, and practicing mindfulness—can boost general vitality, health, and energy levels. When integrating healthy habits into their everyday lives, women may maintain motivation and accountability by creating a support system, defining realistic objectives, and monitoring their progress. Maintaining these healthy behaviors over time and encouraging a beneficial lifestyle shift need consistency and effort.

Overcoming Difficulties and Setbacks: Methods for Maintaining Your Motivation during Your Trip

For women over 40, overcoming obstacles and plateaus is essential to staying motivated and attaining long-term success. Any path toward health and well-being is likely to encounter plateaus and setbacks, which a number of things, such as hormone fluctuations, stress, or changes in lifestyle, may bring on. Women may overcome plateaus and recover momentum in their journey by putting techniques like changing up training routines, making nutritional adjustments, establishing new objectives, and getting guidance from fitness instructors or medical specialists into action. Developing a resilient mentality, engaging in self-compassion exercises, and acknowledging little accomplishments may all help women remain inspired and committed to their wellness and health objectives.

To summarize, maintaining general well-being and attaining long-term success for women over 40 requires managing stress and sleep, developing good habits, and getting beyond obstacles like plateaus and failures. Women may proactively manage their health, maintain a healthy weight, and promote a good and balanced lifestyle as they traverse the many phases of life by placing a high priority on relaxing, implementing sustainable lifestyle adjustments, and keeping a resilient mentality.

For women over 40, maintaining weight reduction via maintenance measures, creating a network of support, and acknowledging personal accomplishments are critical components of long-term well-being and a healthy lifestyle. Adopting efficient maintenance techniques, creating a network of support, and adopting a positive outlook are essential for maintaining weight reduction, advancing general health, and leading a satisfying life free from the obsession with weight, as managing weight may become more challenging as we age.

CHAPTER 5: Embracing Long-Term Wellness

Maintenance Techniques: Maintaining Loss and Avoiding Gain

If women over 40 want to maintain their weight reduction and avoid gaining it back, they must put into practice efficient maintenance measures. In order to assist weight control, this entails implementing a sustainable and balanced meal plan, getting regular exercise, keeping track of your progress, and making lifestyle adjustments. Women may continue to lose weight by keeping a food diary, making reasonable goals, controlling portion sizes, and giving priority to foods high in nutrients. To further promote long-term weight management and general well-being, it is recommended to periodically reevaluate food and activity habits, make any required modifications, and be aware of any obstacles.

The Function of Social Support: Establishing a Community for Ongoing Motivation and Responsibility

Creating a group of support is crucial if women over 40 are to have ongoing responsibility and motivation on their path to health and well-being. Getting involved with friends, family, support groups, or online communities that have similar health and wellness objectives may provide you with a feeling of community, practical counsel, and emotional support. For women looking to maintain their weight loss journey and lead a healthy lifestyle, these strategies can be beneficial in boosting overall well-being, creating a sense of accountability, and sustaining motivation. These strategies include sharing experiences, celebrating milestones, and getting support from a supportive network.

Honoring Your Achievement: Leading a Meaningful and Wellbeing Life Outside of Weight Loss

Before all else, women over 40 should emphasize their holistic well-being and general happiness, which requires them to embrace a rich life beyond weight reduction and celebrate personal triumphs. Prioritizing non-scale achievements like heightened energy, elevated mood, and better general health might assist in changing the emphasis from weight-related objectives to a more comprehensive strategy for total well-being. A satisfying and balanced life may be achieved by following personal interests, making meaningful connections, and doing meaningful activities in addition to focusing on weight control. Further supporting women in leading meaningful and healthy lives and fostering general well-being and happiness include:

- Adopting a good body image
- Engaging in self-compassion exercises
- Cultivating a positive connection with food and exercise

In short, fostering long-term well-being and helping women over 40 have happy lives requires putting maintenance techniques into practice, creating a supportive group, and acknowledging individual accomplishments. Women may maintain their weight reduction efforts, give priority to their general health, and create a whole and happy life that goes beyond obsessing about their weight by adopting a balanced approach to weight management, building a supporting network, and adopting an optimistic outlook.

CONCLUSION

Women's lives continue to unfold with specific experiences, obstacles, and chances for self-discovery and empowerment as they become older, particularly beyond the age of 40. This stage is a great time to embrace the power of self-discovery and empowerment since it often denotes a moment of contemplation, self-renewal, and personal progress. Women who embrace this path may develop a more profound awareness of who they are, what they want, and what they can do, which will eventually help them find contentment, resilience, and a sense of purpose in life.

Accepting Self-Discovery: Examining Individual Passions, Values, and Strengths

A transforming process, embracing self-discovery enables women over 40 to delve into their own beliefs, interests, and talents. Understanding one's identity and purpose may be gained via self-reflection, mindfulness exercises, and meaningful discussions with reliable people. Women may make decisions that are true to themselves and lead to a more purposeful and satisfying existence by identifying their own values and integrating them with their objectives and choices. Discovering one's interests and skills via novel experiences, pastimes, or educational possibilities may enhance personal development and enable women to pursue fulfilling and joyful undertakings.

Promoting Empowerment: Developing Self-Assurance, Adaptability, and Initiative

For women over 40 to develop agency, resiliency, and confidence in overcoming obstacles and achieving their objectives, empowerment is crucial. This entails cultivating an optimistic outlook, establishing attainable objectives, and adopting a growth-oriented viewpoint that recognizes the possibility of ongoing education and individual development. Women may be empowered to overcome barriers, adjust to change, and emerge stronger and more robust by developing resilience through difficulties, setbacks, and life changes. Women may be even more empowered to take charge of their life and boldly pursue their goals and ambitions by developing a feeling of agency by proactive actions, wise choices, and advocacy for their own needs and objectives.

Accepting Personal Development: Promoting Connection, Well-Being, and Mindfulness

Developing meaningful relationships with oneself and others, cultivating general wellbeing, and engaging in mindfulness practices are all components of embracing personal development. Making physical health a priority by engaging in regular exercise, maintaining a healthy diet, and getting enough sleep may promote general vitality and well-being. Meditation, introspection, and thankfulness exercises are effective ways to cultivate mindfulness, which may lead to increased emotional equilibrium, mental clarity, and self-awareness. A full and engaging social life may be fostered by cultivating meaningful ties with encouraging friends, family, and the community. These connections can provide a feeling of belonging, emotional support, and a common purpose.

To sum up, women over 40 embarking on a revolutionary path of self-discovery and empowerment must embrace their own beliefs, interests, and talents; cultivate agency, resilience, and confidence; and nurture relationships, mindfulness, and wellbeing. Women may develop a better awareness of who they are, become more resilient in the face of adversity, and create a meaningful, purpose-driven existence that is in line with their goals and genuine selves by using the power of self-discovery and empowerment.